The Vibrant Dash Diet Meals

The Best Diet With Irresistible Meals For Anyone

Hugh Ward

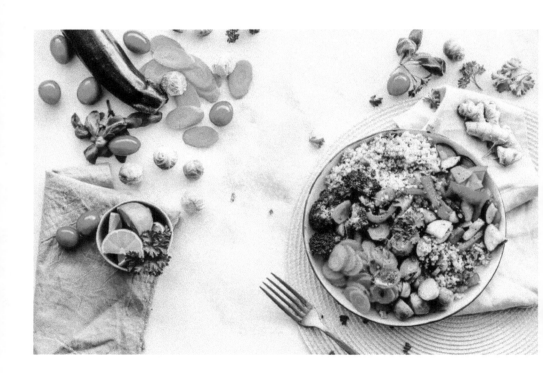

TABLE OF CONTENT

Turkey Sandwich

Preparation time: 10 minutes

Cooking time: 25 minutes

Servings: 4

Ingredients:

- 1 turkey breast, skinless, boneless and sliced into 4 pieces
- 1 eggplant, sliced into 4 slices
- Black pepper to the taste
- 1 tablespoon olive oil
- 1 tablespoon oregano, chopped
- ½ cup low sodium tomato sauce
- ½ cup low-fat cheddar cheese, shredded
- 4 whole wheat bread slices

Directions:

1. Heat up a grill over medium-high heat, add the turkey slices, drizzle half of the oil over them, sprinkle the black pepper, cook for 8 minutes on each side and transfer to a plate.

2. Arrange the eggplant slices on the heated grill, drizzle the rest of the oil over them,

season with black pepper as well, cook them for 4 minutes on each side and transfer to the plate with the turkey slices as well.

3. Arrange 2 bread slices on a working surface, divide the cheese on each, divide the eggplant slices and turkey ones on each, sprinkle the oregano, drizzle the sauce all over and top with the other 2 bread slices.

4. Divide the sandwiches between plates and serve.

Nutrition info per serving: 265 calories, 21.2g protein, 22.1g carbohydrates, 10.6g fat, 6.3g fiber, 47mg cholesterol, 985mg sodium, 572mg potassium

Turkey Tortillas

Preparation time: 10 minutes

Cooking time: 20 minutes

Servings: 4

Ingredients:

- 4 whole wheat tortillas
- ½ cup fat-free yogurt
- 1 pound turkey, breast, skinless, boneless and cut into strips
- 1 tablespoon olive oil
- 1 red onion, sliced
- 1 zucchini, cubed
- 2 tomatoes, cubed
- Black pepper to the taste

Directions:

1. Heat up a pan with the oil over medium heat, add the onion, stir and sauté for 5 minutes.
2. Add the zucchini and tomatoes, toss and cook for 2 minutes more.
3. Add the turkey meat, toss and cook for 13 minutes more.

4. Spread the yogurt on each tortilla, add divide the turkey and zucchini mix, roll, divide between plates and serve.

Nutrition info per serving: 380 calories, 40.4g protein, 31g carbohydrates, 10.5g fat, 4.9g fiber, 86mg cholesterol, 242mg sodium, 730mg potassium

Chicken with Peppers

Preparation time: 10 minutes

Cooking time: 25 minutes

Servings: 4

Ingredients:

- 2 chicken breasts, skinless, boneless and cubed
- 1 red onion, chopped
- 2 tablespoons olive oil
- 1 eggplant, cubed
- 1 red bell pepper, cubed
- 1 yellow bell pepper, cubed
- Black pepper to the taste
- 2 cups coconut milk

Directions:

1. Heat up a pan with the oil over medium-high heat, add the onion, stir and cook for 3 minutes.
2. Add the bell peppers, toss and cook for 2 minutes more.

3. Add the chicken and the other ingredients, toss, bring to a simmer and cook over medium heat for 20 minutes more.
4. Divide everything between plates and serve.

Nutrition info per serving: 524 calories, 25.6g protein, 18.2g carbohydrates, 41.3g fat, 7.7g fiber, 65mg cholesterol, 85mg sodium, 851mg potassium

Balsamic Turkey

Preparation time: 10 minutes

Cooking time: 40 minutes

Servings: 4

Ingredients:

- 1 big turkey breast, skinless, boneless and sliced
- 2 tablespoons balsamic vinegar
- 1 tablespoon olive oil
- 2 garlic cloves, minced
- 1 tablespoon Italian seasoning
- Black pepper to the taste
- 1 tablespoon cilantro, chopped

Directions:

1. In a baking dish, mix the turkey with the vinegar, the oil and the other ingredients, toss, introduce in the oven at 400 degrees F and bake for 40 minutes.
2. Divide everything between plates and serve with a side salad.

Nutrition info per serving: 149 calories, 17.2g protein, 5.2g carbohydrates, 6.2g fat, 0.5g fiber, 45mg cholesterol, 1017mg sodium, 317mg potassium

Cheesy Turkey

Preparation time: 10 minutes

Cooking time: 1 hour

Servings: 4

Ingredients:

- 1 pound turkey breast, skinless, boneless and sliced
- 2 tablespoons olive oil
- 1 cup canned tomatoes, no-salt-added, chopped
- Black pepper to the taste
- 1 cup fat-free cheddar cheese, shredded
- 2 tablespoons parsley, chopped

Directions:

1. Grease a baking dish with the oil, arrange the turkey slices into the pan, spread the tomatoes over them, season with black pepper, sprinkle the cheese and parsley on top, introduce in the oven at 400 degrees F and bake for 1 hour.
2. Divide everything between plates and serve.

Nutrition info per serving: 301 calories, 26.9g protein, 7g carbohydrates, 18.4g fat, 1.2g fiber, 78mg cholesterol, 1330mg sodium, 487mg potassium

Coconut Turkey

Preparation time: 10 minutes

Cooking time: 23 minutes

Servings: 4

Ingredients:

- 1 pound turkey breast, skinless, boneless and cubed
- 1 tablespoon olive oil
- ½ cup low-fat parmesan, grated
- 2 shallots, chopped
- 1 cup coconut milk
- Black pepper to the taste

Directions:

1. Heat up a pan with the oil over medium-high heat, add the shallots, toss and cook for 5 minutes.
2. Add the meat, coconut milk, and black pepper, toss and cook over medium heat for 15 minutes more.
3. Add the parmesan, cook for 2-3 minutes, divide everything between plates and serve.

Nutrition info per serving: 323 calories, 23.4g protein, 9.1g carbohydrates, 22.2g fat, 1.9g fiber, 60mg cholesterol, 1352mg sodium, 533mg potassium

Chicken and Shrimp

Preparation time: 10 minutes

Cooking time: 14 minutes

Servings: 4

Ingredients:

- 1 tablespoon olive oil
- 1 pound chicken breast, skinless, boneless and cubed
- ¼ cup low-sodium chicken stock
- 1 pound shrimp, peeled and deveined
- ½ cup coconut cream
- 1 tablespoon cilantro, chopped

Directions:

1. Heat up a pan with the oil over medium heat, add the chicken, toss and cook for 8 minutes.
2. Add the shrimp and the other ingredients, toss, cook everything for 6 minutes more, divide into bowls and serve.

Nutrition info per serving: 363 calories, 50.6g protein, 3.4g carbohydrates, 15.4g fat, 0.7g fiber,

311mg cholesterol, 348mg sodium, 692mg potassium

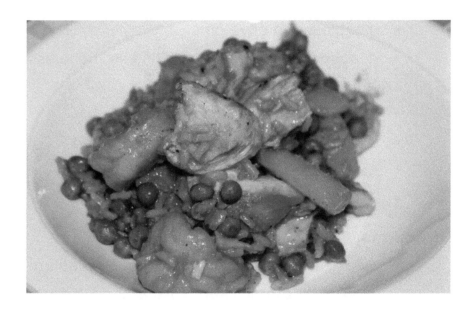

Turkey and Asparagus

Preparation time: 10 minutes

Cooking time: 40 minutes

Servings: 4

Ingredients:

- 1 pound turkey breast, skinless, and cut into strips
- 1 cup coconut cream
- 1 cup low-sodium chicken stock
- 2 tablespoons parsley, chopped
- 1 bunch asparagus, trimmed and halved
- 1 teaspoon chili powder
- 2 tablespoons olive oil
- A pinch of sea salt and black pepper

Directions:

1. Heat up a pan with the oil over medium-high heat, add the turkey and some black pepper, toss and cook for 5 minutes.
2. Add the asparagus, chili powder and the other ingredients, toss, bring to a simmer and cook over medium heat for 30 minutes more.

3. Divide everything between plates and serve.

Nutrition info per serving: 327 calories, 21.9g protein, 9.9g carbohydrates, 23.4g fat, 2.9g fiber, 49mg cholesterol, 1202mg sodium, 591mg potassium

Buttery Cashew Turkey

Preparation time: 10 minutes

Cooking time: 40 minutes

Servings: 4

Ingredients:

- 1 pound turkey breast, skinless, boneless and cubed
- 1 cup cashews, chopped
- 1 yellow onion, chopped
- ½ tablespoon olive oil
- Black pepper to the taste
- ½ teaspoon sweet paprika
- 2 and ½ tablespoons cashew butter
- ¼ cup low-sodium chicken stock
- 1 tablespoon cilantro, chopped

Directions:

1. Heat up a pan with the oil over medium-high heat, add the onion, stir and sauté for 5 minutes.
2. Add the meat and brown it for 5 minutes more.

3. Add the rest of the ingredients, toss, bring to a simmer and cook over medium heat for 30 minutes.
4. Divide the whole mix between plates and serve.

Nutrition info per serving: 401 calories, 26.8g protein, 21.5g carbohydrates, 24.5g fat, 2.5g fiber, 49mg cholesterol, 1168mg sodium, 638mg potassium

Turkey and Cranberries Mix

Preparation time: 10 minutes

Cooking time: 35 minutes

Servings: 6

Ingredients:

- 2 pounds turkey breasts, skinless, boneless and cubed
- 1 tablespoon olive oil
- 1 red onion, chopped
- 1 cup dried cranberries
- 1 cup low-sodium chicken stock
- ¼ cup cilantro, chopped
- Black pepper to the taste

Directions:

1. Heat up a pot with the oil over medium-high heat, add the onion, stir and sauté for 5 minutes.

2. Add the meat, berries and the other ingredients, bring to a simmer and cook over medium heat for 30 minutes more.
3. Divide the mix between plates and serve.

Nutrition info per serving: 272 calories, 26.2g protein, 30.8g carbohydrates, 4.9g fat, 2.5g fiber, 65mg cholesterol, 1558mg sodium, 487mg potassium

Chicken Breast and Tomatoes

Preparation time: 5 minutes

Cooking time: 35 minutes

Servings: 4

Ingredients:

- 1 cup tomatoes, crushed

- 1 teaspoon five spice

- 2 chicken breast halves, skinless, boneless and halved

- 1 tablespoon avocado oil

- 2 tablespoons coconut aminos

- Black pepper to the taste

- 1 tablespoons hot pepper

- 1 tablespoon cilantro, chopped

Directions:

1. Heat up a pan with the oil over medium heat, add the meat and brown it for 2 minutes on each side.
2. Add the tomatoes, five spice and the other ingredients, bring to a simmer and cook over medium heat for 30 minutes.
3. Divide the whole mix between plates and serve.

Nutrition info per serving: 167 calories, 22g protein, 4.8g carbohydrates, 6g fat, 1.7g fiber, 65mg cholesterol, 74mg sodium, 317mg potassium

Turkey and Greens

Preparation time: 10 minutes

Cooking time: 17 minutes

Servings: 4

Ingredients:

- 1 pound turkey breast, boneless, skinless and cubed
- 1 cup mustard greens
- 1 teaspoon nutmeg, ground
- 1 teaspoon allspice, ground
- 1 yellow onion, chopped
- Black pepper to the taste
- 1 tablespoon olive oil

Directions:

1. Heat up a pan with the oil over medium-high heat, add the onion and the meat and brown for 5 minutes.
2. Add the rest of the ingredients, toss, cook over medium heat for 12 minutes more, divide between plates and serve.

Nutrition info per serving: 167 calories, 20.1g protein, 49g carbohydrates, 5.7g fat, 1.8g fiber, 49mg cholesterol, 1156mg sodium, 439mg potassium

Chicken and Almond Mushrooms

Preparation time: 10 minutes

Cooking time: 20 minutes

Servings: 4

Ingredients:

- 2 chicken breasts, skinless, boneless and halved
- ½ pound white mushrooms, halved
- 1 tablespoon olive oil
- 1 cup canned tomatoes, no-salt-added, chopped
- 2 tablespoons almonds, chopped
- 2 tablespoons olive oil
- ½ teaspoon chili flakes
- Black pepper to the taste

Directions:

1. Heat up a pan with the oil over medium-high heat, add the mushrooms, toss and sauté for 5 minutes.

2. Add the meat, toss and cook for 5 minutes more.
3. Add the tomatoes and the other ingredients, bring to a simmer and cook over medium heat for 10 minutes.
4. Divide the mix between plates and serve.

Nutrition info per serving: 206 calories, 23.9g protein, 4.3g carbohydrates, 10.7g fat, 1.5g fiber, 65mg cholesterol, 68mg sodium, 487mg potassium

Chili Chicken

Preparation time: 10 minutes

Cooking time: 20 minutes

Servings: 4

Ingredients:

- 2 red chilies, chopped
- 1 tablespoon olive oil
- 1 yellow onion, chopped
- 1 pound chicken breasts, skinless, boneless and cubed
- 1 cup tomatoes, crushed
- 10 ounces canned artichoke hearts, drained and quartered
- Black pepper to the taste
- ½ cup low-sodium chicken stock
- 2 tablespoons lime juice

Directions:

1. Heat up a pan with the oil over medium heat, add the onion and the chilies, stir and sauté for 5 minutes.
2. Add the meat, toss and brown for 5 minutes more.

3. Add the rest of the ingredients, bring to a simmer over medium heat and cook for 10 minutes.
4. Divide the mix between plates and serve.

Nutrition info per serving: 299 calories, 36g protein, 11.9g carbohydrates, 12.1g fat, 5g fiber, 101mg cholesterol, 185mg sodium, 689mg potassium

Chives Chicken and Beets

Preparation time: 10 minutes

Cooking time: 0 minutes

Servings: 4

Ingredients:

- 1 carrot, shredded

- 2 beets, peeled and shredded

- ½ cup avocado mayonnaise

- 1 cup smoked chicken breast, skinless, boneless, cooked and shredded

- 1 teaspoon chives, chopped

Directions:

1. In a bowl, combine the chicken with the beets and the other ingredients, toss and serve right away.

Nutrition info per serving: 348 calories, 27g protein, 6.5g carbohydrates, 25.6g fat, 1.4g fiber,

105mg cholesterol, 354mg sodium, 202mg potassium

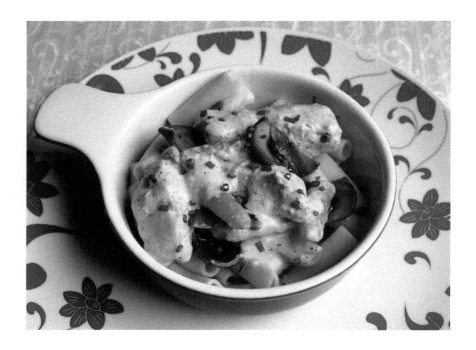

Turkey Salad

Preparation time: 4 minutes

Cooking time: 0 minutes

Servings: 4

Ingredients:

- 2 cups turkey breast, skinless, boneless, cooked and shredded
- 1 cup celery stalks, chopped
- 2 spring onions, chopped
- 1 cup black olives, pitted and halved
- 1 tablespoon olive oil
- 1 teaspoon lime juice
- 1 cup fat-free yogurt

Directions:

1. In a bowl, combine the turkey with the celery and the other ingredients, toss and serve cold.

Nutrition info per serving: 187 calories, 17.7g protein, 12g carbohydrates, 7.3g fat, 1.7g fiber,

30mg cholesterol, 1198mg sodium, 245mg potassium

Chicken with Tomatoes and Grapes

Preparation time: 10 minutes

Cooking time: 40 minutes

Servings: 4

Ingredients:

- 1 carrot, cubed

- 1 yellow onion, sliced

- 1 tablespoon olive oil

- 1 cup tomatoes, cubed

- ¼ cup low-sodium chicken stock

- 2 garlic cloves, chopped

- 1 pound chicken thighs, skinless and boneless

- 1 cup green grapes

- Black pepper to the taste

Directions:

1. Grease a baking pan with the oil, arrange the chicken thighs inside and add the other ingredients on top.
2. Bake at 390 degrees F for 40 minutes, divide between plates and serve.

Nutrition info per serving: 289 calories, 33.9g protein, 10.3g carbohydrates, 12.1g fat, 1.7g fiber, 101mg cholesterol, 120mg sodium, 521mg potassium

Turkey and Barley

Preparation time: 5 minutes

Cooking time: 55 minutes

Servings: 4

Ingredients:

- 1 tablespoon olive oil

- 1 turkey breast, skinless, boneless and sliced

- Black pepper to the taste

- 2 celery stalks, chopped

- 1 red onion, chopped

- 2 cups low-sodium chicken stock

- ½ cup barley

- 1 teaspoon lemon zest, grated

- 1 tablespoon lemon juice

- 1 tablespoon chives, chopped

Directions:

1. Heat up a pot with the oil over medium-high heat, add the meat and the onion, toss and brown for 5 minutes.
2. Add the celery and the other ingredients, toss, bring to a simmer, reduce heat to medium, simmer for 50 minutes, divide into bowls and serve.

Nutrition info per serving: 194 calories, 15.5g protein, 23.3g carbohydrates, 4.1g fat, 4.8g fiber, 25mg cholesterol, 796mg sodium, 195mg potassium

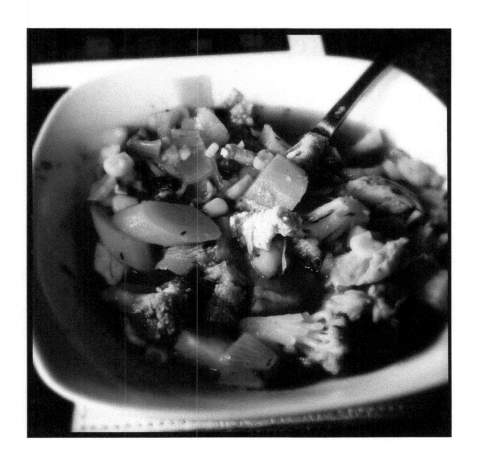

Turkey with Radishes

Preparation time: 10 minutes

Cooking time: 35 minutes

Servings: 4

Ingredients:

- 1 turkey breast, skinless, boneless and cubed

- 2 red beets, peeled and cubed

- 1 cup radishes, cubed

- 1 red onion, chopped

- ¼ cup low-sodium chicken stock

- Black pepper to the taste

- 1 tablespoon olive oil

- 2 tablespoon chives, chopped

Directions:

1. Heat up a pan with the oil over medium-high heat, add the meat and the onion, toss and brown for 5 minutes.

2. Add the beets, radishes and the other ingredients, bring to a simmer and cook over medium heat for 30 minutes more.
3. Divide the mix between plates and serve.

Nutrition info per serving: 124 calories, 10.6g protein, 10.9g carbohydrates, 4.6g fat, 2.4g fiber, 23mg cholesterol, 605mg sodium, 427mg potassium

Paprika Pork Mix

Preparation time: 10 minutes

Cooking time: 45 minutes

Servings: 8

Ingredients:

- 2 pounds pork meat, boneless and cubed

- 1 red onion, chopped

- 1 tablespoon olive oil

- 3 garlic cloves, minced

- 1 cup low-sodium beef stock

- 2 tablespoons sweet paprika

- Black pepper to the taste

- 1 tablespoon chives, chopped

Directions:

1. Heat up a pan with the oil over medium heat, add the onion and the meat, toss and brown for 5 minutes.

2. Add the rest of the ingredients, toss, reduce heat to medium, cover and cook for 40 minutes.
3. Divide the mix between plates and serve.

Nutrition info per serving: 199 calories, 22.8g protein, 2.6g carbohydrates, 10g fat, 1g fiber, 75mg cholesterol, 104mg sodium, 66mg potassium

Pork and Carrots

Preparation time: 10 minutes

Cooking time: 30 minutes

Servings: 4

Ingredients:

- 1 pound pork stew meat, cubed

- ¼ cup low-sodium vegetable stock

- 2 carrots, peeled and sliced

- 2 tablespoons olive oil

- 1 red onion, sliced

- 2 teaspoons sweet paprika

- Black pepper to the taste

Directions:

1. Heat up a pan with the oil over medium heat, add the onion, stir and sauté for 5 minutes.

2. Add the meat, toss and brown for 5 minutes more.

3. Add the rest of the ingredients, bring to a simmer and cook over medium heat for 20 minutes.
4. Divide the mix between plates and serve.

Nutrition info per serving: 328 calories, 34g protein, 6.4g carbohydrates, 18.1g fat, 1.8g fiber, 98mg cholesterol, 98mg sodium, 596mg potassium

Cilantro Pork

Preparation time: 10 minutes

Cooking time: 35 minutes

Servings: 4

Ingredients:

- 2 red onions, sliced

- 2 green onions, chopped

- 1 tablespoon olive oil

- 2 teaspoons ginger, grated

- 4 pork chops

- 3 garlic cloves, chopped

- Black pepper to the taste

- 1 carrot, chopped

- 1 cup low sodium beef stock

- 2 tablespoons tomato paste, low sodium

- 1 tablespoon cilantro, chopped

Directions:

1. Heat up a pan with the oil over medium heat, add the green and red onions, toss and sauté them for 3 minutes.
2. Add the garlic and the ginger, toss and cook for 2 minutes more.
3. Add the pork chops and cook them for 2 minutes on each side.
4. Add the rest of the ingredients, bring to a simmer and cook over medium heat for 25 minutes more.
5. Divide the mix between plates and serve.

Nutrition info per serving: 332 calories, 19.9g protein, 10.1g carbohydrates, 23.6g fat, 2.3g fiber, 69mg cholesterol, 11mg sodium, 528mg potassium

Coriander Pork

Preparation time: 10 minutes

Cooking time: 45 minutes

Servings: 4

Ingredients:

- ½ cup low-sodium beef stock
- 2 tablespoons olive oil
- 2 pounds pork stew meat, cubed
- 1 teaspoon coriander, ground
- 2 teaspoons cumin, ground
- Black pepper to the taste
- 1 cup cherry tomatoes, halved
- 4 garlic cloves, minced
- 1 tablespoon cilantro, chopped

Directions:

1. Heat up a pan with the oil over medium heat, add the garlic and the meat, toss and brown for 5 minutes.

2. Add the stock and the other ingredients, bring to a simmer and cook over medium heat for 40 minutes.
3. Divide everything between plates and serve.

Nutrition info per serving: 559 calories, 67.4g protein, 10.1g carbohydrates, 3.2g fat, 29.3g fiber, 195mg cholesterol, 156mg sodium, 988mg potassium

Balsamic Pork

Preparation time: 10 minutes

Cooking time: 20 minutes

Servings: 4

Ingredients:

- 2 tablespoons balsamic vinegar

- 1/3 cup coconut aminos

- 1 tablespoon olive oil

- 4 ounces mixed salad greens

- 1 cup cherry tomatoes, halved

- 4 ounces pork stew meat, cut into strips

- 1 tablespoon chives, chopped

Directions:

1. Heat up a pan with the oil over medium heat, add the pork, coconut aminos and the vinegar, toss and cook for 15 minutes.

2. Add the salad greens and the other ingredients, toss, cook for 5 minutes more, divide between plates and serve.

Nutrition info per serving: 125 calories, 9.1g protein, 6.8g carbohydrates, 6.4g fat, 0.6g fiber, 24mg cholesterol, 49mg sodium, 269mg potassium

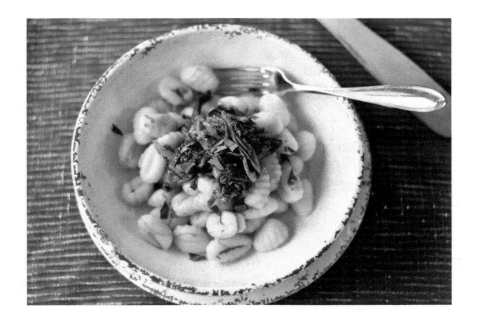

Cilantro Pork Skillet

Preparation time: 10 minutes

Cooking time: 25 minutes

Servings: 4

Ingredients:

- 1 pound pork butt, trimmed and cubed
- 1 tablespoon olive oil
- 1 yellow onion, chopped
- 3 garlic cloves, minced
- 1 tablespoon thyme, dried
- 1 cup low-sodium chicken stock
- 2 tablespoons low-sodium tomato paste
- 1 tablespoon cilantro, chopped

Directions:

1. Heat up a pan with the oil over medium-high heat, add the onion and the garlic, toss and cook for 5 minutes.
2. Add the meat, toss and cook for 5 more minutes.

3. Add the rest of the ingredients, toss, bring to a simmer, reduce heat to medium and cook the mix for 15 minutes more.
4. Divide the mix between plates and serve right away.

Nutrition info per serving: 274 calories, 36.6g protein, 5.3g carbohydrates, 11.2g fat, 1.2g fiber, 104mg cholesterol, 104mg sodium, 484mg potassium

Pork and Zucchinis

Preparation time: 10 minutes

Cooking time: 30 minutes

Servings: 4

Ingredients:

- 2 pounds pork loin boneless, trimmed and cubed

- 2 tablespoons avocado oil

- ¾ cup low-sodium vegetable stock

- ½ tablespoon garlic powder

- 1 tablespoon marjoram, chopped

- 2 zucchinis, roughly cubed

- 1 teaspoon sweet paprika

- Black pepper to the taste

Directions:

1. Heat up a pan with the oil over medium-high heat, add the meat, garlic powder and the marjoram, toss and cook for 10 minutes.

2. Add the zucchinis and the other ingredients, toss, bring to a simmer, reduce heat to medium and cook the mix for 20 minutes more.
3. Divide everything between plates and serve.

Nutrition info per serving: 359 calories, 61.1g protein, 5.7g carbohydrates, 9.1g fat, 2.1g fiber, 166mg cholesterol, 166mg sodium, 1289mg potassium

Nutmeg Pork

Preparation time: 10 minutes

Cooking time: 8 hours

Servings: 4

Ingredients:

- 3 tablespoons olive oil

- 2 pounds pork shoulder roast

- 2 teaspoons sweet paprika

- 1 teaspoon garlic powder

- 1 teaspoon onion powder

- 1 teaspoon nutmeg, ground

- 1 teaspoon allspice, ground

- Black pepper to the taste

- 1 cup low-sodium vegetable stock

Directions:

1. In your slow cooker, combine the roast with the oil and the other ingredients, toss, put the lid on and cook on Low for 8 hours.

2. Slice the roast, divide it between plates and serve with the cooking juices drizzled on top.

Nutrition info per serving: 689 calories, 38.8g protein, 3.2g carbohydrates, 57.1g fat, 1g fiber, 161mg cholesterol, 187mg sodium, 77mg potassium

Peppercorn Pork

Preparation time: 10 minutes

Cooking time: 35 minutes

Servings: 4

Ingredients:

- 2 pounds pork stew meat, cubed

- 2 tablespoons olive oil

- 1 cup low-sodium vegetable stock

- 1 celery stalk, chopped

- 1 teaspoon black peppercorns

- 2 shallots, chopped

- 1 tablespoon chives, chopped

- 1 cup coconut cream

- Black pepper to the taste

Directions:

1. Heat up a pan with the oil over medium heat, add the shallots and the meat, toss and brown for 5 minutes.

2. Add the celery and the other ingredients, toss, bring to a simmer and cook over medium heat for 30 minutes more.
3. Divide everything between plates and serve right away.

Nutrition info per serving: 690 calories, 68.2g protein, 5.7g carbohydrates, 43.3g fat, 1.8g fiber, 195mg cholesterol, 182mg sodium, 1077mg potassium

Parsley Pork and Tomatoes

Preparation time: 10 minutes

Cooking time: 30 minutes

Servings: 4

Ingredients:

- 2 garlic cloves, minced

- 2 pounds pork stew meat, ground

- 2 cups cherry tomatoes, halved

- 1 tablespoon olive oil

- Black pepper to the taste

- 1 red onion, chopped

- ½ cup low-sodium vegetable stock

- 2 tablespoons low-sodium tomato paste

- 1 tablespoon parsley, chopped

Directions:

1. Heat up a pan with the oil over medium heat, add the onion and the garlic, toss and sauté for 5 minutes.
2. Add the meat and brown it for 5 minutes more.
3. Add the rest of the ingredients, toss, bring to a simmer, cook over medium heat for 20 minutes more, divide into bowls and serve.

Nutrition info per serving: 551 calories, 68.2g protein, 8.6g carbohydrates, 25.6g fat, 2.1g fiber, 195mg cholesterol, 163mg sodium, 1131mg potassium

Lemon Pork Chops

Preparation time: 10 minutes

Cooking time: 35 minutes

Servings: 4

Ingredients:

- 4 pork chops
- 2 tablespoons olive oil
- 1 teaspoon smoked paprika
- 1 tablespoon sage, chopped
- 2 garlic cloves, minced
- 1 tablespoon lemon juice
- Black pepper to the taste

Directions:

1. In a baking dish, combine the pork chops with the oil and the other ingredients, toss, introduce in the oven and bake at 400 degrees F for 35 minutes.
2. Divide the pork chops between plates and serve with a side salad.

Nutrition info per serving: 322 calories, 18.2g protein, 1.2g carbohydrates, 27.1g fat, 0.5g fiber, 69mg cholesterol, 57mg sodium, 304mg potassium

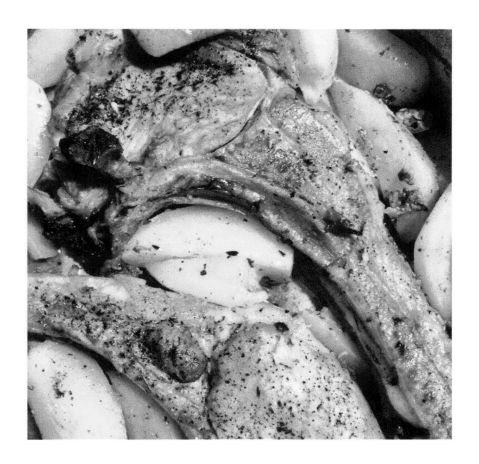

Coconut Pork Mix

Preparation time: 10 minutes

Cooking time: 30 minutes

Servings: 4

Ingredients:

- 1 pound pork stew meat, cubed
- 1 eggplant, cubed
- 1 tablespoon coconut aminos
- 1 teaspoon five spice
- 2 garlic cloves, minced
- 2 Thai chilies, chopped
- 2 tablespoons olive oil
- 2 tablespoons low-sodium tomato paste
- 1 tablespoon cilantro, chopped
- ½ cup low-sodium vegetable stock

Directions:

1. Heat up a pan with the oil over medium-high heat, add the garlic, chilies and the meat and brown for 6 minutes.
2. Add the eggplant and the other ingredients, bring to a simmer and cook over medium heat for 24 minutes.

3. Divide the mix between plates and serve.

Nutrition info per serving: 348 calories, 35.1g protein, 10.5g carbohydrates, 18.2g fat, 4.5g fiber, 98mg cholesterol, 134mg sodium, 711mg potassium

Lime Pork

Preparation time: 10 minutes

Cooking time: 30 minutes

Servings: 4

Ingredients:

- 2 tablespoons lime juice
- 4 scallions, chopped
- 1 pound pork stew meat, cubed
- 2 garlic cloves, minced
- 2 tablespoons olive oil
- Black pepper to the taste
- ½ cup low-sodium vegetable stock
- 1 tablespoon cilantro, chopped

Directions:

1. Heat up a pan with the oil over medium heat, add the scallions and the garlic, toss and cook for 5 minutes.
2. Add the meat, toss and cook for 5 minutes more.
3. Add the rest of the ingredients, bring to a simmer and cook over medium heat for 20 minutes.

4. Divide the mix between plates and serve.

Nutrition info per serving: 310 calories, 33.7g protein, 2.1g carbohydrates, 18g fat, 0.6g fiber, 98mg cholesterol, 87mg sodium, 490mg potassium

Coriander Pork

Preparation time: 10 minutes

Cooking time: 30 minutes

Servings: 4

Ingredients:

- 1 red onion, sliced
- 1 pound pork stew meat, cubed
- 2 red chilies, chopped
- 2 tablespoons balsamic vinegar
- ½ cup coriander leaves, chopped
- Black pepper to the taste
- 2 tablespoons olive oil
- 1 tablespoon low-sodium tomato sauce

Directions:

1. Heat up a pan with the oil over medium heat, add the onion and the chilies, toss and cook for 5 minutes.
2. Add the meat, toss and cook for 5 minutes more.
3. Add the rest of the ingredients, toss, bring to a simmer and cook over medium heat for 20 minutes more.

4. Divide everything between plates and serve right away.

Nutrition info per serving: 323 calories, 34g protein, 4.9g carbohydrates, 18.1g fat, 1.1g fiber, 98mg cholesterol, 91mg sodium, 566mg potassium

Basil Pork Mix

Preparation time: 10 minutes

Cooking time: 36 minutes

Servings: 4

Ingredients:

- 2 tablespoons olive oil
- 2 spring onions, chopped
- 1 pound pork chops
- 2 tablespoons basil pesto
- 1 cup cherry tomatoes, cubed
- 2 tablespoons low-sodium tomato paste
- ½ cup parsley, chopped
- ½ cup low-sodium vegetable stock
- Black pepper to the taste

Directions:

1. Heat up a pan with the olive oil over medium-high heat, add the spring onions and the pork chops, and brown for 3 minutes on each side.
2. Add the pesto and the other ingredients, toss gently, bring to a simmer and cook over medium heat for 30 minutes more.

3. Divide everything between plates and serve.

Nutrition info per serving: 446 calories, 26.9g protein, 4.8g carbohydrates, 35.4g fat, 1.4g fiber, 98mg cholesterol, 110mg sodium, 579mg potassium

Pork and Tomatoes

Preparation time: 10 minutes

Cooking time: 1 hour

Servings: 4

Ingredients:

- 1 green bell pepper, chopped
- 1 red bell pepper, chopped
- 1 yellow bell pepper, chopped
- 1 red onion, chopped
- 1 pound pork chops
- 1 tablespoon olive oil
- Black pepper to the taste
- 26 ounces canned tomatoes, no-salt-added and chopped
- 2 tablespoons parsley, chopped

Directions:

1. Grease a roasting pan with the oil, arrange the pork chops inside and add the other ingredients on top.
2. Bake at 390 degrees F for 1 hour, divide everything between plates and serve.

Nutrition info per serving: 459 calories, 28.3g protein, 14.9g carbohydrates, 32.3g fat, 4.3g fiber, 98mg cholesterol, 93mg sodium, 1038mg potassium

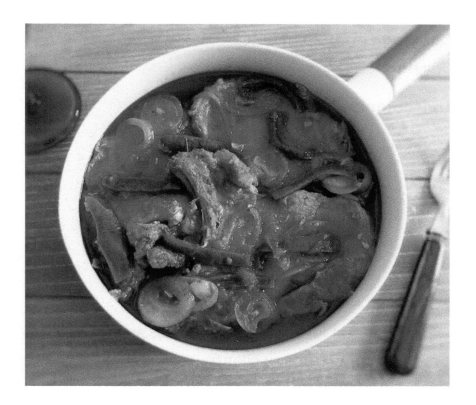

Lamb and Cherry Tomatoes Mix

Preparation time: 10 minutes

Cooking time: 25 minutes

Servings: 4

Ingredients:

- 1 tablespoon olive oil
- 1 red onion, chopped
- 1 cup cherry tomatoes, halved
- 1 pound lamb stew meat, ground
- 1 tablespoon chili powder
- Black pepper to the taste
- 2 teaspoons cumin, ground
- 1 cup low-sodium vegetable stock
- 2 tablespoons cilantro, chopped

Directions:

1. Heat up the a pan with the oil over medium-high heat, add the onion, lamb and chili powder, toss and cook for 10 minutes.
2. Add the rest of the ingredients, toss, cook over medium heat for 15 minutes more.

3. Divide into bowls and serve.

Nutrition info per serving: 275 calories, 33.2g protein, 6.8g carbohydrates, 12.5g fat, 2.1g fiber, 102mg cholesterol, 145mg sodium, 617mg potassium

Pork with Green Beans

Preparation time: 10 minutes

Cooking time: 35 minutes

Servings: 4

Ingredients:

- 1 pound pork stew meat, cubed
- 1 cup radishes, cubed
- ½ pound green beans, trimmed and halved
- 1 yellow onion, chopped
- 1 tablespoon olive oil
- 2 garlic cloves, minced
- 1 cup canned tomatoes, no-salt-added and chopped
- 2 teaspoons oregano, dried
- Black pepper to the taste

Directions:

1. Heat up a pan with the oil over medium-high heat, add the onion and the garlic, toss and cook for 5 minutes.
2. Add the meat, toss and cook for 5 minutes more.

3. Add the rest of the ingredients, bring to a simmer and cook over medium heat for 25 minutes.
4. Divide everything into bowls and serve.

Nutrition info per serving: 316 calories, 35.3g protein, 10.3g carbohydrates, 14.8g fat, 3.9g fiber, 98mg cholesterol, 85mg sodium, 777mg potassium

Lamb with Scallions and Mushrooms

Preparation time: 10 minutes
Cooking time: 40 minutes
Servings: 4

Ingredients:

- 1 pound lamb shoulder, boneless and cubed
- 8 white mushrooms, halved
- 2 tablespoons olive oil
- 1 yellow onion, chopped
- 2 garlic cloves, minced
- 1 an ½ tablespoons fennel powder
- Black pepper to the taste
- A bunch of scallions, chopped
- 1 cup low-sodium vegetable stock

Directions:

1. Heat up a pan with the oil over medium heat, add the onion and the garlic, toss and cook for 5 minutes.
2. Add the meat and the mushrooms, toss and cook for 5 minutes more.

3. Add the other ingredients, toss, bring to a simmer and cook over medium heat for 30 minutes.
4. Divide the mix into bowls and serve.

Nutrition info per serving: 298 calories, 33.7g protein, 5.4g carbohydrates, 15.5g fat, 1.3g fiber, 102mg cholesterol, 126mg sodium, 581mg potassium

Pork with Tomatoes and Spinach

Preparation time: 10 minutes

Cooking time: 30 minutes

Servings: 4

Ingredients:

- 1 pound pork, ground
- 2 tablespoons olive oil
- 1 red onion, chopped
- ½ pound baby spinach
- 4 garlic cloves, minced
- ½ cup low-sodium vegetable stock
- ½ cup canned tomatoes, no-salt-added, chopped
- Black pepper to the taste
- 1 tablespoon chives, chopped

Directions:

1. Heat up a pan with the oil over medium-high heat, add the onion and the garlic, toss and cook for 5 minutes.

2. Add the meat, toss and brown for 5 minutes more.
3. Add the rest of the ingredients except the spinach, toss, bring to a simmer, reduce heat to medium and cook for 15 minutes.
4. Add the spinach, toss, cook the mix for another 5 minutes, divide everything into bowls and serve.

Nutrition info per serving: 257 calories, 32.1g protein, 7g carbohydrates, 11.3g fat, 2.3g fiber, 83mg cholesterol, 130mg sodium, 918mg potassium

Warm Pork Salad

Preparation time: 10 minutes

Cooking time: 15 minutes

Servings: 4

Ingredients:

- 2 cups baby spinach
- 1 pound pork steak, cut into strips
- 1 tablespoon olive oil
- 1 cup cherry tomatoes, halved
- 2 avocados, peeled, pitted and cut into wedges
- 1 tablespoon balsamic vinegar
- ½ cup low-sodium vegetable stock

Directions:

1. Heat up a pan with the oil over medium-high heat, add the meat, toss and cook for 10 minutes.
2. Add the spinach and the other ingredients, toss, cook for 5 minutes more, divide into bowls and serve.

Nutrition info per serving: 544calories, 31.9g protein, 11.5g carbohydrates, 42.1g fat, 7.7g fiber, 108mg cholesterol, 116mg sodium, 1066mg potassium

Chili Pork and Apples

Preparation time: 10 minutes

Cooking time: 40 minutes

Servings: 4

Ingredients:

- 2 pounds pork stew meat, cut into strips
- 2 green apples, cored and cut into wedges
- 2 garlic cloves, minced
- 2 shallots, chopped
- 1 tablespoon sweet paprika
- ½ teaspoon chili powder
- 2 tablespoons avocado oil
- 1 cup low-sodium chicken stock
- Black pepper to the taste
- A pinch of red chili pepper flakes

Directions:

1. Heat up a pan with the oil over medium heat, add the shallots and the garlic, toss and sauté for 5 minutes.
2. Add the meat and brown for another 5 minutes.

3. Add the apples and the other ingredients, toss, bring to a simmer and cook over medium heat for 30 minutes more.
4. Divide everything between plates and serve.

Nutrition info per serving: 561calories, 67.6g protein, 18.3g carbohydrates, 23.3g fat, 3.8g fiber, 195mg cholesterol, 174mg sodium, 1062mg potassium

Hot Pork Chops

Preparation time: 10 minutes

Cooking time: 1 hour and 10 minutes

Servings: 4

Ingredients:

- 4 pork chops
- 2 tablespoons olive oil
- 2 garlic cloves, minced
- ¼ cup low-sodium vegetable stock
- 1 tablespoon cinnamon powder
- Black pepper to the taste
- 1 teaspoon chili powder
- ½ teaspoon onion powder

Directions:

1. In a roasting pan, combine the pork chops with the oil and the other ingredients, toss, introduce in the oven and bake at 390 degrees F for 1 hour and 10 minutes.
2. Divide the pork chops between plates and serve with a side salad.

Nutrition info per serving: 323calories, 18.3g protein, 1.4g carbohydrates, 27g fat, 0.3g fiber, 69mg cholesterol, 72mg sodium, 35mg potassium

Creamy Pork Chops

Preparation time: 10 minutes

Cooking time: 20 minutes

Servings: 4

Ingredients:

- 2 tablespoons olive oil
- 4 pork chops
- 1 yellow onion, chopped
- 1 tablespoon chili powder
- 1 cup coconut milk
- ¼ cup cilantro, chopped

Directions:

1. Heat up a pan with the oil over medium-high heat, add the onion and the chili powder, toss and sauté for 5 minutes.
2. Add the pork chops and brown them for 2 minutes on each side.
3. Add the coconut milk, toss, bring to a simmer and cook over medium heat for 11 minutes more.
4. Add the cilantro, toss, divide everything into bowls and serve.

Nutrition info per serving: 471calories, 19.9g protein, 7g carbohydrates, 41.5g fat, 2.6g fiber, 69mg cholesterol, 86mg sodium, 514mg potassium

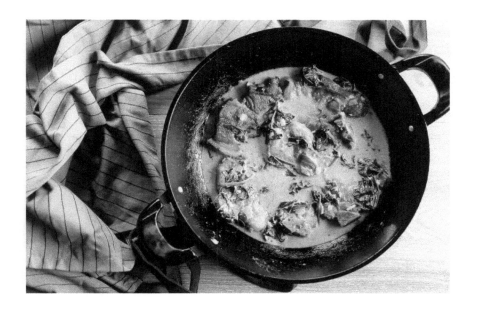

Pork with Paprika Peaches

Preparation time: 10 minutes

Cooking time: 25 minutes

Servings: 4

Ingredients:

- 2 pounds pork tenderloin, roughly cubed
- 2 peaches, stones removed and cut into quarters
- ¼ teaspoon onion powder
- 2 tablespoons olive oil
- ¼ teaspoon smoked paprika
- ¼ cup low-sodium vegetable stock
- Black pepper to the taste

Directions:

1. Heat up a pan with the oil over medium heat, add the meat, toss and cook for 10 minutes.
2. Add the peaches and the other ingredients, toss, bring to a simmer and cook over medium heat for 15 minutes more.

3. Divide the whole mix between plates and serve.

Nutrition info per serving: 416calories, 60.2g protein, 7.4g carbohydrates, 15.2g fat, 1.3g fiber, 166mg cholesterol, 138mg sodium, 1110mg potassium

Lamb and Radish Skillet

Preparation time: 10 minutes

Cooking time: 35 minutes

Servings: 4

Ingredients:

- ½ cup low-sodium vegetable stock
- 1 pound lamb stew meat, cubed
- 1 cup radishes, cubed
- 1 tablespoon cocoa powder
- Black pepper to the taste
- 1 yellow onion, chopped
- 1 tablespoon olive oil
- 2 garlic cloves, minced
- 1 tablespoon parsley, chopped

Directions:

1. Heat up a pan with the oil over medium-high heat, add the onion and the garlic, toss and sauté for 5 minutes.
2. Add the meat, toss and brown for 2 minutes on each side.

3. Add the stock and the other ingredients, toss, bring to a simmer and cook over medium heat for 25 minutes more.
4. Divide everything between plates and serve.

Nutrition info per serving: 265calories, 32.8g protein, 5.4g carbohydrates, 12.1g fat, 1.6g fiber, 102mg cholesterol, 117mg sodium, 549mg potassium

Pork and Lemon Artichokes Mix

Preparation time: 10 minutes

Cooking time: 25 minutes

Servings: 4

Ingredients:

- 2 pounds pork stew meat, cut into strips
- 2 tablespoons avocado oil
- 1 tablespoon lemon juice
- 1 tablespoon lemon zest, grated
- 1 cup canned artichokes, drained and cut into quarters
- 1 red onion, chopped
- 2 garlic cloves, minced
- ½ teaspoon chili powder
- Black pepper to the taste
- 1 teaspoon sweet paprika
- 1 jalapeno, chopped
- ¼ cup low-sodium vegetable stock
- ¼ cup rosemary, chopped

Directions:

1. Heat up a pan with the oil over medium-high heat, add the onion and the garlic, toss and sauté for 4 minutes.
2. Add the meat, artichokes, chili powder, the jalapeno and the paprika, toss and cook for 6 minutes more.
3. Add the rest of the ingredients, toss, bring to a simmer and cook over medium heat for 15 minutes more.
4. Divide the whole mix into bowls and serve.

Nutrition info per serving: 544calories, 68.6g protein, 12.1g carbohydrates, 23.7g fat, 6.7g fiber, 195mg cholesterol, 176mg sodium, 1117mg potassium

Parmesan Pork and Sauce

Preparation time: 10 minutes

Cooking time: 20 minutes

Servings: 4

Ingredients:

- 2 pounds pork stew meat, roughly cubed
- 1 cup cilantro leaves
- 4 tablespoons olive oil
- 1 tablespoon pine nuts
- 1 tablespoon fat-free parmesan, grated
- 1 tablespoon lemon juice
- 1 teaspoon chili powder
- Black pepper to the taste

Directions:

1. In a blender, combine the cilantro with the pine nuts, 3 tablespoons oil, parmesan and lemon juice and pulse well.
2. Heat up a pan with the remaining oil over medium heat, add the meat, chili powder

and the black pepper, toss and brown for 5 minutes.

3. Add the cilantro sauce, and cook over medium heat for 15 minutes more, stirring from time to time.

4. Divide the pork between plates and serve right away.

Nutrition info per serving: 622calories, 67.1g protein, 0.9g carbohydrates, 37.8g fat, 0.4g fiber, 196mg cholesterol, 162mg sodium, 903mg potassium

Pork with Mango and Tomatoes

Preparation time: 10 minutes

Cooking time: 25 minutes

Servings: 4

Ingredients:

- 2 shallots, chopped
- 2 tablespoons avocado oil
- 1 pound pork stew meat, cubed
- 1 mango, peeled and roughly cubed
- 2 garlic cloves, minced
- 1 cup tomatoes, and chopped
- Black pepper to the taste
- ½ cup basil, chopped

Directions:

1. Heat up a pan with the oil over medium heat, add the shallots and the garlic, toss and cook for 5 minutes.
2. Add the meat, toss and cook for 5 minutes more.

3. Add the rest of the ingredients, toss, bring to a simmer and cook over medium heat for 15 minutes more.
4. Divide the mix into bowls and serve.

Nutrition info per serving: 315calories, 34.7g protein, 16.1g carbohydrates, 12.3g fat, 2.3g fiber, 98mg cholesterol, 71mg sodium, 727mg potassium

Pork and Sweet Potatoes

Preparation time: 10 minutes

Cooking time: 35 minutes

Servings: 4

Ingredients:

- 1 red onion, cut into wedges
- 2 sweet potatoes, peeled and cut into wedges
- 4 pork chops
- 1 tablespoon rosemary, chopped
- 1 tablespoon lemon juice
- 2 teaspoons olive oil
- Black pepper to the taste
- 2 teaspoons thyme, chopped
- ½ cup low-sodium vegetable stock

Directions:

1. In a roasting pan, combine the pork chops with the potatoes, onion and the other ingredients and toss gently.
2. Bake at 400 degrees F for 35 minutes, divide everything between plates and serve.

Nutrition info per serving: 335calories, 18.9g protein, 13.7g carbohydrates, 22.5g fat, 2.5g fiber, 69mg cholesterol, 63mg sodium, 635mg potassium

Cilantro Pork and Chickpeas

Preparation time: 10 minutes

Cooking time: 25 minutes

Servings: 4

Ingredients:

- 1 pound pork stew meat, cubed

- 1 cup canned chickpeas, no-salt-added, drained

- 1 yellow onion, chopped

- 1 tablespoon olive oil

- Black pepper to the taste

- 10 ounces canned tomatoes, no-salt-added and chopped

- 2 tablespoons cilantro, chopped

Directions:

1. Heat up a pan with the oil over medium-high heat, add the onion, toss and sauté for 5 minutes.
2. Add the meat, toss and cook for 5 minutes more.
3. Add the rest of the ingredients, toss, simmer over medium heat for 15 minutes, divide everything into bowls and serve.

Nutrition info per serving: 476calories, 43.8g protein, 35.7g carbohydrates, 17.6g fat, 10.2g fiber, 98mg cholesterol, 84mg sodium, 1073mg potassium

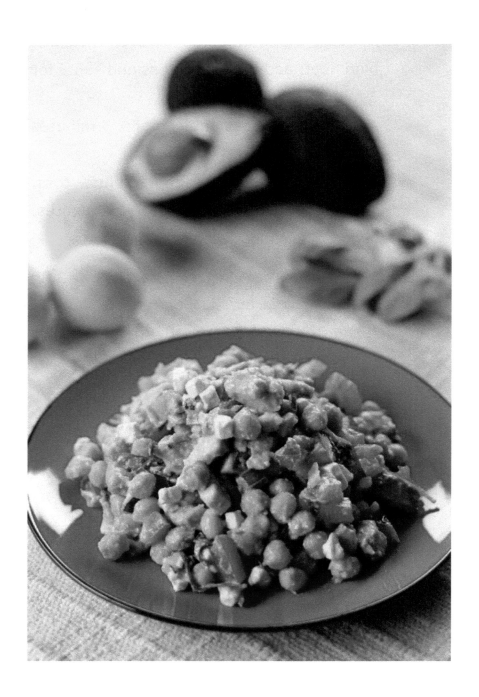